AF881012

Stop Hiding Your Smile!

A Parent's Guide to
Confidently Choosing
an Orthodontist

Dustin S. Burleson, D.D.S.

Wasteland Press
www.wastelandpress.net
Shelbyville, KY USA

Stop Hiding Your Smile!
A Parent's Guide to Confidently Choosing an Orthodontist
by Dustin S. Burleson, D.D.S.

Copyright © 2011 Dustin S. Burleson, D.D.S.
ALL RIGHTS RESERVED

First Printing – October 2011
ISBN: 978-1-60047-627-3

NO PART OF THIS BOOK MAY BE REPRODUCED IN ANY FORM, BY PHOTOCOPYING OR BY ANY ELECTRONIC OR MECHANICAL MEANS, INCLUDING INFORMATION STORAGE OR RETRIEVAL SYSTEMS, WITHOUT PERMISSION IN WRITING FROM THE COPYRIGHT OWNER/AUTHOR

Printed in the U.S.A.

0 1 2 3 4 5 6 7

Table of Contents

INTRODUCTION:
The Top-5 Reasons People Avoid Seeing the Orthodontist

My name is Dr. Dustin Burleson, and I'm an orthodontist!

When people I hear what I do for a living, they almost automatically… wince! They try not to be too obvious about it. (Hey, orthodontists have feelings, too!) But it's usually there, if only for a brief moment.

It's okay; I'm used to it. The fact is, the less you know about orthodontics, the more reason you have to be afraid of it. Once upon a time, orthodontists meant one thing: heavy, ugly, tight and painful metal braces.

They were hard to put on, hard to keep on and painful to remove. They meant avoiding certain foods and even activities for a long, long time. Many people still cling to the unfounded notion that all braces are created equal; and are performed the same way they were back in 1982!

The fact of the matter is that orthodontics is more than just braces. How much more? Technically speaking, orthodontics is the specialty of dentistry devoted to building beautiful smiles by bringing teeth, lips and jaws into proper alignment.

Straight teeth simply function better, are easier to clean and are more likely to last your lifetime. Properly aligned jaws may reduce the risk of jaw joint dysfunction (TMJ). Orthodontics is a wonderful investment with life-long returns, and yet people still fear sending their child to the orthodontist for one simple reason: **fear of pain**!

In fact, the one recurring theme I hear about folks going to the orthodontist is that it's going to hurt. (Short answer, it doesn't!) But there are lots of other fears that keep people from coming to see me and my colleagues.

What are some of them and, what's more, how many of them are there? I will say that, in my experience, the following are *The Top-5 Reasons People Avoid Seeing the Orthodontist*:

1. **Patients are afraid it's going to hurt.** Pain is the number one reason most people avoid going to the orthodontist. In fact, modern technology – and choosing the right orthodontist! – can ensure that your child enjoys a pain-free orthodontist experience.

2. **Patients are afraid it's going to cost too much.** Not only are most orthodontic procedures more affordable than ever, but insurance, payment plans and a variety of other financing options make this all but a moot point for most of my patients. Remember, orthodontists aren't in this to get rich; they're here to make sure that your child's teeth, smile and jaw are aligned to make his or her life better – period! We're not going to let something like price get in the way of creating a better, safer, healthier smile for your child.

3. **Patients are afraid it's going to take too long / miss too much school or work.** Regardless of the type of orthodontic procedure your child needs, time is of the essence. Modern technology and ease of access allows us to work around your child's school schedule with a minimum of absences. After initial visits and barring the actual procedure itself, most visits and/or adjustments are routine and can take anywhere from 15 to 45 minutes.

4. **Patients do not see the need to take action.** Eroding, crooked or unaligned smiles can take time to happen, but the time to act is now. Orthodontic irregularities don't just heal on their own or "go away" if you ignore them. Your child's

smile and his overall dental health are too important to ignore out of questions of pain, convenience or even price.

5. **Patients have been treated in the past with an attitude of indifference.** Let's face it, not all doctors are created equal. Every profession has its "bad apples," and to say dentistry is the exception would be to write fiction instead of fact. There is no room for indifference when it comes to your child's healthcare. Find an orthodontic specialist that offers not only state of the art technological advances to your child, but state of the art service as well. Orthodontic specialists know what it's like to sit in the chair, and should provide every opportunity for patients, especially our younger patients, to feel comfortable, safe and secure in our care.

If you've shared any of these concerns, hopefully this brief discussion has put your mind at ease. But don't stop now; there's much more to explore here. In my practice, I see parents like you every day. You're worried about your child's teeth, but none too eager to put him or her through a painful, costly procedure that may take them out of school for hours or even days at a time.

But we see children as well; children that are self-conscious about their crooked teeth, who have taken to hiding their smiles to avoid others seeing their mouths, even if the misalignment is minor.

This book is called *Stop Hiding Your Smile* because there is simply no reason for your child not to have a straight, clean, easy to care for, confident and healthy smile! The world of modern orthodontics is not what it was when you or I grew up and had painful, cold, sterile and metal braces.

What you and your child need aren't more questions, but answers. You don't need more doubts, you need results. Well, you've come to the right place. I'm an orthodontist and I'm here to help.

What do I do?

How do I do it?

When should you come see me?

I'm glad you asked: my best patients are active participants in their healthcare decisions. Providing your child with a beautiful smile is an important investment. The time and effort you spend researching orthodontics now will lead to a confident decision in the type of care you receive and when you receive it. Simply stated, **effort equals result**. Be an active participant in your child's healthcare now and reap the rewards for a lifetime.

This short book is meant as a guide for parents who are unfamiliar with orthodontics. Maybe you never had braces as a child, but you want to provide this important investment for your children. Like any unfamiliar endeavor, the initial steps can be overwhelming. Giving you the confidence to make decisions about the timing of your child's orthodontic treatment is the basic goal of this publication.

In fact, this book answers **over two dozen of the most commonly asked questions about orthodontics**. *Stop Hiding Your Smile* is easy to read and will serve as a quick reference and valuable resource in the journey of improving your child's smile.

PART 1

Finding an Orthodontic Specialist

Question # 1:
Why is My Child's Smile So Important?

The First Reason Your Child's Smile is So Important: *Health*

The fact is, a **straight smile** is a **healthy smile**. Like anything else in life, balance is all about proportion. Straight teeth and jaws that align mean the rest of the mouth and, indeed, face can grow proportionally, ensuring good oral health.

First and foremost, I am a dentist and a specialist who deals specifically with making sure your child has the healthiest mouth possible. This includes such possible orthodontic treatment as:

Braces for children
Invisalign or clear tooth aligners
Keyless Expanders to improve jaw alignment
Habit appliances to prevent side-effects from thumb sucking
Space maintainers to help permanent teeth erupt into alignment
Retainers to prevent unwanted crowding
Functional appliances to improve facial balance
Early treatment and growth modification
Customized appliances designed uniquely for each patient
Soft Tissue Laser for optimal gum tissue esthetics

While it may seem like an exhaustive list, the fact is your child may only need braces, or appliances; rarely both. The bottom line is, health comes first, last and always! But keep reading, there are lots more reasons why a healthy smile is an important smile:

The Second Reason Your Child's Smile is So Important: *Confidence*

Why go to the trouble of seeing a specialist for your child's smile? Simple: so she can stop hiding it! Have you noticed your child hiding her smile more often lately? Has she become less secure around you, her siblings, her friends, at school?

It can be easy for you as the parent to overlook the irregularities in your child's smile, or to see crooked teeth or even an overbite as "cute." True, all children are beautiful in their parents' eyes but the fact remains, crooked or overly-spaced teeth can present real obstacles for your child's confidence level now, as well as later in life.

Having a clean, healthy and straight smile gives your child the confidence he needs to stop hiding his smile – and start showing it off instead. Do your child a favor and talk to him about his smile, and how it might be affecting him.

What's more, look at your child objectively for the following signs that he may be in need of a qualified orthodontist:

Early or late loss of teeth
Difficulty in chewing or biting
Mouth breathing
Finger sucking or other oral habits
Crowding, misplaced, or blocked-out teeth
Jaws that shift, make sounds, protrude or retrude
Speech difficulty
Biting the cheek or into the roof of the mouth
Protruding teeth
Teeth that meet in an abnormal way or don't meet at all
Facial imbalance
Grinding or clenching of teeth

Such signs are an indication that you should visit an orthodontist sooner rather than later.

The Third Reason Your Child's Smile is So Important: *Socialization*

Let's face it: kids can be cruel! From elementary school on, and sometimes even sooner if your child is involved in Pre-K, peer groups and classmates look for any reason to tease, ostracize or even outright humiliate kids who are perceived as "different."

While I'm not condoning such behavior, I see it every day when my patients come in complaining of the other kids teasing them about their crooked teeth, buck teeth or overbite. The fact is, they may not share this with you, for fear of being even more embarrassed at home as well as school.

You might be surprised what your kids will tell me while sitting in my chair that they won't tell you while sitting at the dinner table. A straight, clean and healthy smile can not only give your child the confidence she needs to embrace her true worth, but can also pave the way toward easier socialization at school, at church, in groups and during extracurricular activities.

The Fourth Reason Your Child's Smile is So Important: *Comfort*

Headaches.
Toothaches.
Sinus problems.
Dry mouth.
Snoring.
Drooling.

Bad breath.
Insomnia.

All of these and much more are symptoms of a smile that isn't straight, jaws that aren't aligned or teeth that are too close together – or not quite close enough. Oftentimes, however, the mouth is the last place we check for signs of discomfort, loss of sleep, or even a simple headache.

If your child's pediatrician can't figure out why she's not sleeping well or experiencing headaches or even insomnia for which there seems to be no cause, a simple 30-minute exam at your local orthodontist could provide a clear solution in no time!

The Fifth Reason Your Child's Smile is So Important: *Proper Development*

Picture your child like a giant, living, breathing, walking, talking puzzle. As he or she grows, more and more of the puzzle falls into place over time. The expectation, of course, is that all of the pieces of the puzzle fit perfectly.

And, usually, it does. His arms and legs grow proportionally so that he can run, jump, skip and bend with ease. His eyes and nose and smile form at about the same time, so that his face is in proportion.

Teeth, tongue, lips, smile should all grow in proportion as well. But when it doesn't, that's where the problems start. Now imagine your child's smile as a piece of that puzzle we first talked about.

What might happen if his or her mouth doesn't quite "fit"? The fact is, the sooner you straighten your child's smile, the faster it will develop as it should; straight, clean and healthy!

The Sixth Reason Your Child's Smile is So Important: *Peace of Mind*

As a parent, I know you want the best for your child. No parent wants their child to suffer, either from teeth that actually hurt, from headaches you can't explain, insomnia that affects everything else or insecurity your child may be feeling because of a crooked or oversized smile.

The fact is, your child's formative years are actually the most sensitive for his or her teeth. Now is the time to pay close attention to your child's smile, his behavior, his peer relationships, even his confidence level.

If any or all are lacking, a qualified orthodontist can give you and your child the peace of mind you both crave.

Parting Words About Why Your Child's Smile is So Important

I probably didn't need to tell you most of this. As a parent, no doubt you want the best for your child, including his or her smile. But hopefully this chapter has solidified how important early, safe and expert help can be to ensuring a bright smile for your child – as well as a bright future!

Question # 2:
Why Should I Choose a Specialist for My Child's Orthodontic Care?

The fact of the matter is that your child may or may not need a specialist for his or her dental needs. The question within a question becomes, "How will you *know* if your child needs a specialist or not?"

Before we explore the additional question of whether or not your child needs to see a specialist, let's be clear on what, exactly, an orthodontist is:

What An Orthodontist Does

Orthodontists are **dental specialists** who have completed 2-3 years of additional education beyond dental school to learn the proper way to align teeth and jaws. This further training qualifies your orthodontist to **identify**, **diagnose** and more importantly **treat** a broad spectrum of dental irregularities your family dentist may not, such as:

Early or late loss of teeth
Difficulty in chewing or biting
Crowding, misplaced, or blocked-out teeth
Jaws that shift, make sounds, protrude or retrude
Speech difficulty
Biting the cheek or into the roof of the mouth
Protruding teeth
Teeth that meet in an abnormal way or don't meet at all
Facial imbalance
Grinding or clenching of teeth

The nature of some of these issues, many of which present themselves in early to late childhood or adolescence, grow increasingly serious with lack of proper treatment. Having a specialist identify, diagnose and treat such ailments is the # 1 reason for seeing an orthodontist.

What Your Orthodontist *Doesn't* Do

From what your orthodontist does, let's shift to what he or she *doesn't* do. For instance, your orthodontist doesn't do fillings or cleanings. He or she exclusively provides orthodontic and dentofacial orthopedic treatment to help shape the jaws and teeth into dazzling smiles.

This begs the question, are orthodontists dentists? Yes, actually, they are. In fact, **all orthodontists *are* dentists**, but **only 6% of dentists are orthodontists**.

So, why should I choose a specialist for my child's orthodontic care?

Some problems simply need a specialist's care. When you're pregnant, you go to an obstetrician. When you have stomach problems beyond what your general practitioner is qualified to handle, you visit your gastroenterologist.

Well, in the same way that pediatricians or obstetricians are medical specialists, orthodontists are **dental specialists**. When you choose an orthodontist, you are choosing a specialist with the broadest experience and training possible.

Unique treatment requirements and otherwise difficult bite problems are common, everyday scenarios for your orthodontist. In the interest of receiving the most efficient and effective orthodontic treatment possible, choose an orthodontic specialist.

How do I know my doctor is an orthodontist?

One question I get asked frequently is "How do I know if my doctor is an orthodontist?" It's a good question, and a critical one to ask as you seek additional treatment for your child's dental issues.

Here's the answer: Only orthodontists can belong to the American Association of Orthodontists (AAO). If you're looking for a local orthodontist, go on-line and visit www.braces.org to find a specialist in your area. This FREE website features not only a searchable database of orthodontists but educational tips, answers and resources to help you on your quest for your child's healthiest smile!

Or you can simply ask your doctor if he or she has completed a 2-3 year residency in orthodontics and check with your state dental board to follow-up on his reply. Dentists and orthodontists in most states will be registered differently with the dental board.

Do your homework; be a "dental detective" while on the hunt for such vital information. Look for the words "dental specialist in orthodontics" or ask your general dentist for a referral to a specialist. In urban and suburban areas, it will take minimal effort to find a specialist.

In more remote rural locations, your search might take you to another city or town. Don't be afraid to ask your dentist if an orthodontist travels to your town every month to see patients.

There's a chance an orthodontist from a larger city comes to your town and works out of another dental office once or twice per month. Looking around can save valuable driving time and money.

Question # 3:
How Early in Life Should My Child See the Orthodontist?

Is six years too young to go to the orthodontist?

Is ten years too "old"?

You're not alone if this is the first question that comes to mind after your dentist recommends your first-grader visit the orthodontist. In fact, one of the most common questions I'm asked, almost on a daily basis, is **how young** is **too young** for one's child to go to the orthodontist.

First and foremost, let's set the record straight on when your child should first visit the orthodontist. The definitive, debate-ending answer is **seven years of age**. Period; end of story.

Why so early?

The answer is simple: age seven is the earliest time your orthodontist can determine future jaw and tooth alignment. Prior to this time, the final position of the jaws and teeth is just a guess. An educated guess, perhaps, but a guess nonetheless.

So before seven is too young, physically speaking. What about too old? Is there even such a thing? Actually, there is. Case in point: waiting to take your child to the orthodontist until they are 12 or 13, however, can be very risky.

Let me explain why: at the age of seven, your child's upper and lower permanent front teeth are developing. These teeth set the stage for future jaw position and serious problems can develop if they come into the wrong position.

I meet a lot of parents who say to me, "I don't believe in early orthodontics." This is like saying you don't believe in the sun. You can hide from it, pretend it's not there or refuse to acknowledge it, but the simple fact remains. If you're not aware of the potential risks, you can get burnt.

Do you really want to risk future damage tomorrow by burying your head in the sand today?

What these parents are really saying is, "It doesn't make sense to me why we would do anything until all of the baby teeth are gone." After all, they reason in the same breath, "I didn't get my braces until high school and I was just fine."

Now, don't get me wrong; I'm not here to harp on parents or name names. In fact, both of these statements are valid concerns and both can actually be true.

Nine times out of ten, the orthodontic exam for a seven year old is just that; an exam. The orthodontic exam at age seven rules out possible problems at this young age and allows the orthodontist to monitor the growth and development of the teeth and jaws until your child is ready for braces. At this stage, your orthodontist can hopefully point out potential "problem spots" and now you can both be aware of them during regular and routine follow-up visits.

For one out of ten seven-year-old patients, however, interceptive orthodontics can prevent a variety of potentially dangerous issues before they become more severe, including:

- **Serious jaw alignment problems;**
- **Impacted teeth;**
- **Chipped or fractured teeth;**
- **Gum tissue recession;**
- **Even teasing at school and other problems that are much more expensive and much more difficult to correct later.**

The exam at age seven is important for your peace of mind and for your child's well being. Don't miss it. It's a critical step in your journey toward a beautiful new smile for your son or daughter.

Question # 4:
What Signs Should I be Looking for Before Seeing an Orthodontist?

If you are concerned about your child's smile, regardless of his or her age, consider the following: the research is clear on several treatment problems that arise early in life.

These are significant findings as early as age seven that can significantly impact future jaw and tooth alignment and there are no excuses why early treatment shouldn't start immediately.

If your child is suffering from any, several or all of the following early indicators, consider having them addressed by an orthodontic specialist sooner rather than later:

- **Crossbites:** A "crossbite" occurs when the jaw is deviating to one side with an improper fit of the upper and lower teeth from left to right or front to back. Crossbites can lead to worn and chipped teeth, jaw pain and asymmetric growth of the jaws. Left untreated, the crossbite will require more-extensive treatment later in life, and significant jaw surgery in the most-severe examples.
- **Thumb-sucking:** Thumb-sucking habits beginning at the age of seven or older should be corrected immediately in order to prevent severe jaw and tooth alignment problems.
- **Miscellaneous concerns:** There are several associated issues that you should also be looking for as soon as your child turns seven, to include the following:

    - Permanent teeth that are growing into the wrong spot;

- o Severely protruded front teeth at risk for injury or causing teasing at school, and....
- o Severe crowding with permanent teeth erupting into poor-quality gum tissue are all reasons to intervene early.

Waiting will have very serious consequences, often requiring more treatment and higher cost later in life. What most parents fail to realize is that these treatment problems are urgent and should be treated as such.

So, what if your child does not have one of these urgent problems we just discussed? Then it is important to weigh and consider your options for early treatment versus waiting for braces when all of the permanent teeth are in place. Listen for key concepts such as spacing and crowding, overbite or overjet and the anticipated impact of the treatment on the face.

Your orthodontist will explain these concepts in easy-to-understand terms and help you decide what the best time for treatment is in your particular case. Remember, this is your child, your money, your decision. The orthodontist is a highly-trained professional in a position to help your child, but he or she should not make the final decision in your healthcare.

Emotional Concerns Can Be Just as Traumatic as Physical Issues

Pain isn't the only reason your child may be suffering as a result of a crooked, unhealthy or unsightly smile. Some dental irregularities can be relatively painless, physically speaking, but certainly damaging to your child's confidence levels.

Like it or not, your child's peer groups, even his or her "friends," can be overtly insensitive when it comes to his or her appearance. Even well-meaning buddies or BFFs can unintentionally wound a child's fragile ego with so-called "harmless" nicknames that refer to your child's overbite, crooked teeth or smile.

Going from grade school to middle school with nicknames like "Bucky" or "Toothy" following him or her is only going to make your child's confidence suffer as new teachers are met, new friendships are formed and new social pressures are introduced.

If you are nervous about the appearance of your child's teeth or if your child is self-conscious of his or her appearance, early treatment might be the best investment you ever make in your child's future.

On the other hand, if you are comfortable with crooked teeth for a little longer and your child has no desire or is not mature enough to take care of the braces, then waiting is a perfect option, provided you visit the orthodontist every 6-12 months for growth evaluations and monitoring for the perfect time to start braces.

Do not assume that your child who did not need early treatment at age seven still doesn't need any intervention at age nine or 10. This false assumption can cost you valuable time and money later in your child's life.

My recommendation? See the orthodontist regularly even if you know your child won't need braces for several years. Starting treatment at the best time is a satisfying job for parents, saving both time and money.

PART 2

Fixing the Right Things at the Right Time

Question # 5:
What Will Happen at the Initial Consultation?

Many questions surround your first visit to a new orthodontist, not the least of which is the subject of this particular chapter: *What will happen at the initial consultation?*

To answer this very common question, and perhaps several others you might not even realize you need answering yet, let me walk you through the typical first office visit, from the initial appointment forward: Your first appointment is scheduled following your initial phone call to your orthodontist's office.

The receptionist – who often also doubles as your scheduler – will work with you to find the perfect time for an optimal visit, taking into account not only the orthodontist's schedule but also your schedule as well as your child's. Following this phone call a packet of information will be sent to you with information about your orthodontist's office and the examination appointment. (A health history and map will usually be enclosed.)

During the first appointment several important things will typically happen. You will be greeted by someone who is generally referred to as the "treatment coordinator." She will review your personal information, health history, and your chief concerns with your teeth and/or smile. Your orthodontist will then conduct a thorough examination of your face, mouth, teeth, and jaws to determine whether you can benefit from orthodontic treatment and, if so, when treatment should begin.

Your orthodontist will answer as many questions as possible. If you had additional questions, personal questions or need follow-up questions, there are often a variety of ways to get those questions answered for you. (See next section for several great tips on where – and how – to find answers.)

Any qualified orthodontist wanting to stay competitive and loyal to his or her patients should have a state of the art computer program that can simulate and demonstrate many things about orthodontic treatment. If orthodontic treatment is recommended now, he or she may proceed and take diagnostic records.

In order for the doctor to accurately diagnose your problems and plan your treatment, some additional information is needed beyond what is found during the examination. The doctor will request diagnostic records that can sometimes be done the day of the examination or will ask you to return so the office can have a complete set of records to evaluate your needs.

Your orthodontist will typically take molds of your teeth at this point, from which plaster replicas are made, digital photographs of your face and teeth, x-rays of your teeth and surrounding bone, and a headfilm x-ray to evaluate the position of the jaw structures.

At the consultation your doctor will fully explain the nature and extent of your needs and an individualized plan of treatment. This appointment is important because it is your time to have all questions answered and feel comfortable with the orthodontic treatment plan.

Your treatment coordinator will review costs of treatment and payment arrangements. Usually, your orthodontist will request about 20% of the total fee when treatment begins and the remainder is divided into monthly payments for the duration of treatment. (Special arrangements can often be made for those needing assistance; be sure to speak with your treatment coordinator beforehand.)

What happens next? Well, the next couple of appointments will be dedicated to placing your braces. You will also receive individual instruction in hygiene, diet and appliance care from our hygiene specialists. Once the braces are placed, subsequent adjustment visits are scheduled every six to eight weeks. These visits normally take between 15-45 minutes.

Question # 6:
What if I Still Have Questions after the Initial Consultation?

It's very common for parents and their children to have additional questions beyond the initial consultation. Between the anxiety of setting up the visit to sitting in an orthodontist's chair to the variety of preliminary and post-visit issues that have to be dealt with, it's easy to get overwhelmed. That's why modern orthodontists make it extremely simple for you to get the answers you need in a way that's simplest for you.

Where to Get Your Questions Answered

Here are just some of the ways you can get your questions answered in your way – and right on time:

Your orthodontist's website: Your orthodontist's website should feature a variety of patient resources including full explanations of every procedure, an interactive map with driving directions, links to the doctor's blog, an FAQ section and several ways to get in touch with the office if you don't find what you're looking for.

Your treatment coordinator: You will usually be assigned a patient contact person – we call this person a "treatment coordinator" in our office – with whom to schedule appointments, confer with rescheduling and, of course, answer any and all questions you may have. In some cases this may literally be the office receptionist or the dental care technician who assisted your orthodontist. More and more offices are assigning patient care representatives who are merely there for support, interaction and, of course, to answer you and your child's questions.

A 24-hour recording: Many orthodontists have modernized their most popular FAQs (or Frequently Asked Questions), most frequently found on their websites or in the office brochure, into a 24-hour recording for their patients' convenience.

The follow-up visit: As we read in the previous chapter, there are a variety of follow-up visits between 15- and 45-minutes in duration depending on the procedure your child is getting. These are wonderful opportunities to either a.) ask questions you may have missed the first time or b.) get further details from your orthodontist him- or herself.

Braces.org: The website of the American Association of Orthodontists offers a wide range of articles and patient information for your records prior to and during orthodontic treatment. The orthodontist locator is a popular feature to help you find a specialist close to home. Remember, only orthodontists can belong to the American Association of Orthodontists, so when you visit www.braces.org you know you're receiving accurate, state-of-the-art information regarding tooth and jaw alignment.

Regardless of how many questions you have, or your comfort level with technology, phone calls or in-person visits, your orthodontist should offer an option that fits your schedule and makes all your unresolved issues crystal clear.

How to Get Your Questions Answered

Now that we know where to get your most burning orthodontic questions answered, here are some simple tips I've amassed over the years to help you easily and effectively get the information you need:

Make a list: The easiest way to get what you want is to know it in advance. Make a list of the various questions you have so that you can quickly and easily go down the list to assure you've got the right answers for the right questions.

Bring it with you: Take the list with you when you go for your child's orthodontist visit. This way you have the questions at hand at the right place at the right time. If you're calling in to get answers, you can also have the list ready and tick off one question for every answer you receive.

Record the answers: If your orthodontist – or his receptionist – speaks too fast or you can't keep up while writing the answers down, why not record them. Your cell phone likely has a "record" feature and, if not, there are many affordable micro-recorders on the market today.

Double-check: Finally, make sure you have the right answer by double-checking with your orthodontist, his or her receptionist or assistant, your answer liaison or simply by Googling your question online!

Knowing where to find the information you need is only half the battle; follow these tips and you'll know how to get what you're looking for as well.

Question # 7:
When is the Best Time to get Braces?

I mentioned in Part 1 the importance of the initial exam at age seven. If your child is above the age of seven and you haven't seen the orthodontist for an initial examination, put this book down immediately and call your orthodontist to schedule the exam today. Really. If you have completed the initial examination, continue to see the orthodontist as scheduled so that he or she can monitor your child's growth. Many is the time I see a pre-teen or early teen in my chair and think to myself, "If only his parents had come to me sooner, he could have avoided lengthier and more-complicated treatment!" For the uninitiated, "lengthier and more-complicated treatment" translate into more expensive orthodontic care for you and your family budget.

Will my child actually need braces at seven?

In the same breath I use to inform parents of the initial exam at age seven, I also mention that most children **will not need braces until 11-13 years of age**. To understand why, you must first know a little bit about the history of orthodontic treatment in the United States. (Stick with me here, folks; it's worth it!)

In the 1960s and 70s, we rarely treated younger children because the technology rarely afforded us the opportunity to align the teeth and jaws without removing teeth. Nearly 80% of children in the previous generation of orthodontic patients had teeth removed and the teeth that were almost always removed do not show up in the mouth until age 11-12. Therefore, nearly everyone who needed braces didn't get them until they were at least 12 years old.

In the 1980s, space age technology made its way to the orthodontist's office in the form of "memory wires," otherwise known as Nickel Titanium alloys. These wires were lighter, gentler and more exciting than anything that had come along in orthodontics in decades. In combination with expansion of the jaws, these memory wires could be used in an entirely new group of patients – younger children aged between seven and 10 years of age.

Suddenly, every child in fourth grade had braces. Our hope in treating more children early was to prevent the removal of permanent teeth later in life or to make the correction of the bite easier or shorter in duration.

Instead of going through a single round of braces at the age of 12 or 13, usually involving the removal of four permanent premolar teeth, patients and orthodontists were getting started earlier and more often in the pursuit of a perfect bite, beautiful smile and the ultimate goal of **no removal of teeth**.

With nearly 30 years of early treatment results in the literature, orthodontists began to ask the question, "Does early treatment always make a difference?" When a well-designed research study at the University of North Carolina was finally completed after 10 years in the making, orthodontists and patients alike were left scratching their heads. All these years, we had been preaching the benefits of early treatment for a majority of our patients and the research ultimately concluded something neither of us had expected: maybe we were being *too* cautious.

In the final analysis, patients with similar bites who waited until they were 11-13 to start treatment had nearly identical results as the patients who started early and avoided two rounds of braces. Confused yet? You're not alone. Parents in every corner of the country are puzzled when they receive different opinions regarding early treatment from several specialists.

So, who is right: the orthodontist who **tells you to wait** or the orthodontist who **recommends you start early**? It depends on your comfort level with the risks involved with waiting in certain cases.

If you were to ask me, I would always recommend that better safe than sorry. Early evaluation allows you the freedom of choice, the luxury of time and the peace of mind knowing that your child's smile is in good hands at the best possible time!

Question # 8:
What if my Child is Nervous About Getting Braces?

Parenting is always a challenge. There is so much to consider, so many questions to answer, so many challenges to face. It can be simple to overlook one more tiny detail in the avalanche of daily brushfires, dilemmas, carpool and permission slips modern parents have to deal with.

The fact of the matter is that when you see your child's face, often the only thing you see is your child's smiling face. That is to say you see the beauty, the charm, the personality, the love and the joy that your child's smile represents.

As parents, we're not taught to look for our children's flaws; we're taught to see the beauty in everything our child does. But the fact of the matter is, the more closely you look at your child's smile – even the more critically you look at your child's smile – the more help you'll be giving them later in life.

That's because today's tiny flaw, crooked tooth, overbite or underbite could be just the thing that contributes to your child's insecurities tomorrow. We all grew up regretting something about our appearance. Perhaps it was our nose, our ears, our gangly arms or spindly legs.

Often we grow out of such awkwardness as our bodies grown and morph and bring things into perspective. But with our smiles, the more we grow the more whatever irregularities we may have as children tend to only grow more pronounced; not less.

Getting braces *will* affect your child's self-confidence. In the short term, the act of physically wearing braces – depending on the style, make and duration – may make your child feel less confident.

Braces still carry a certain stigma around them, which is often unavoidable given the fact that kids often like to make fun of whatever, or whoever, is currently "different."

But the typical duration of braces is much shorter than it used to be when you and I were growing up, so that negative stigma will only last for a brief, short while. (And with clear braces or Invisalign, perhaps not at all!)

However, not getting braces may affect your child's confidence level for much, much longer. With each passing year, over- and underbites can become more pronounced, teeth move out of alignment, not in and what was once a minor issue in childhood becomes a growing concern in adolescence and young adulthood.

Even as parents continue to see their children's imperfections as lovable and adorable, the kids themselves can often dwell on those very same imperfections to the point of insecurity, lack of confidence and even an unwillingness to go out and socialize.

While every child IS beautiful, I'm here to attest to the fact that not every child feels beautiful. I treat children every day who complain of being teased or even bullied at school because of their appearance, and with something as preventable as crooked teeth or a simple over- or underbite, why take the chance?

Tips for Helping Your Child Adjust to Life with Braces

- **All the cool kids are doing it (or soon will be):** Braces are a very popular appliance during the middle school and high school years. Rather than focus on how he or she feels wearing braces, encourage your child to begin actively looking for other kids who are wearing braces. Chances are, they'll find lots more than they ever imagined!

- **Even famous people do it:** Gwen Stefani. Prince Harry. Drew Barrymore. Tom Cruise. Dakota Fanning. Danny Glover. The list of famous people who've worn braces – many of them as adults – could fill half this book. Share with your child how even the most famous people sometimes need a little help through braces.

- **Fast forward:** Many orthodontists provide a "before and after" consultant's session, much like a plastic surgeon. Digital pictures are often used to portray what the child's teeth might look like once the braces have been removed. Have your child focus on the after when he or she gets down about the "before" shots!

- **Be prepared:** Finally, create a "master list" of things your child likes to do; things that make him feel special, confident, brave, calm, relaxed or excited. If you notice him feeling down, consult your list and make plans to do something special in the near future to boost his confidence level back to where you know it belongs!

Question # 9:
Why are we waiting? The teeth look crooked to me!

It's no secret that I'm a big supporter of early evaluation. In fact, in our office, we want to see EVERYONE for an exam by the age of seven. This way we don't miss critical points in development.

However, despite insisting on early visits, I've never been a fan of doing a procedure just for procedure's sake. In fact, only a small percentage of those younger patients who do receive early visits actually require early treatment, in my experience.

As orthodontists, our goal is to achieve both a great smile and a healthy bite. We place special emphasis on interceptive and preventive measures for children.

The timing of treatment is very important in obtaining an ideal result and preventing future problems with tooth and jaw alignment. Periodic evaluations allow the doctor to determine how and when best to treat your child's particular needs.

Assessment of facial growth and supervision of eruption of permanent teeth helps to achieve results, which may otherwise be unattainable if treatment were initiated after the jaws have completed growth.

Some problems are best corrected when the patient is young and may be recommended with the objective of addressing problems before they develop into bigger ones, obtaining better jaw balance, and allowing room for eruption of permanent teeth. Treatment at the ideal time will save you time and money and help prevent tooth or jaw problems before they become more difficult and more expensive to fix.

A critical part of achieving this goal is proper timing in placing your braces. A Pre-Orthodontics Guidance Program allows the orthodontist to time your treatment so that you will have your braces on the shortest amount of time possible to achieve a beautiful result and wise investment.

Early treatment has now been proven through systematic reviews of the literature and prospective, randomized clinical trials (the gold standard in research) to be beneficial for:

- **Crossbites**
- **Underbites**
- **Thumb sucking habits**
- **Early loss of baby teeth**
- **Impacted permanent teeth**
- **Patients with upper front teeth that stick so far forward they are at risk for injury (severe buck teeth)**
- **Patients who are being teased at school due to the appearance of their teeth**
- **Some patients with cleft lip and palate who require jaw expansion prior to surgery**

Everyone else, who may be experiencing crooked teeth and/or moderate overbites, they can typically wait until they are 11-12 to start orthodontic treatment and get the same result... with less time and money invested.

Remember, a consultation doesn't necessarily have to mean a resulting procedure. Many times, as I've indicated, an early visit means just that; a visit. Only infrequently do children as young as 7, 8 or even 9 or 10 need to be treated with a formal procedure.

So if that's what's been keeping you from taking your child to his or her orthodontist early, perhaps now I've allayed some of that fear and you can feel free to schedule that appointment today!

What are the goals of waiting and watching?

Following the initial examination, if you child is not ready for orthodontic treatment, periodic evaluations allow your doctor to determine how and when best to treat your child's particular needs. Assessment of facial growth and supervision of eruption of permanent teeth helps to achieve results, which may otherwise be unattainable if treatment were initiated after the jaws have completed growth.

Some problems are best corrected when the patient is young and may be recommended with the objective of addressing problems before they develop into bigger ones, obtaining better jaw balance, and allowing room for eruption of permanent teeth. Treatment at the ideal time will save you time and money and help prevent tooth or jaw problems before they become more difficult and more expensive to fix.

The overriding goal of treatment in your orthodontist's office is to reduce the length of time that you will have your braces on. Every orthodontist I know prides him- or herself on having the shortest treatment times possible. Thanks to modern technology and the latest in dental procedures, I think you'll be pleasantly surprised by how your orthodontist will be able to complete your orthodontic correction much faster than what is commonly anticipated.

A critical part of achieving this goal is proper timing in placing your braces. Your doctor's Pre-Orthodontics Guidance Program – he or she may call it something else – allows your orthodontist to time your treatment so that you will have your braces on the shortest amount of time possible to achieve a beautiful result and wise investment. Plan on seeing the orthodontic specialist every 6 or 12 months until your child is ready for braces. Often, there is no charge for this periodic evaluation and you can gain peace of mind, knowing your child's teeth and jaws are developing as anticipated in preparation for orthodontic treatment at the perfect time.

PART 3

Focusing on a Plan that is Right for You

Question # 10:
What are the Treatment Options When My Child is Ready?

If your child is ready for orthodontic care, one of the first discussions to have with your orthodontist is which procedure is right for him or her; the options might be much more plentiful than you ever imagined.

If you're like most people, you associate orthodontists with braces, but these days that is just one arm of what I or any orthodontist does. Here are some of the services most orthodontists will provide their patients with during the course of routine treatment:

Metal tie-free braces
Lingual braces placed behind your teeth
Invisalign clear removable aligners
Clear braces
Expanders to match jaw size and tooth size
Habit appliances to eliminate thumb sucking
Space maintainers
Retainers to prevent crowding and shifting of teeth
Headgear to help correct jaw alignment
Functional appliances to help improve facial balance
Early treatment and growth modification
Customized appliances designed uniquely for each patient

While many of these services may seem self-explanatory to you, several will probably not. In the course of the next few questions, I will try to elaborate on several of them, including:

Crossbite Correction
Invisalign
Invisalign Teen
Metal Braces
Clear Braces
Incognito by 3M

Question # 11:
What is a Crossbite? (And Should I Worry if My Child Has One?)

As your child's teeth begin to grow in, there is a LOT more at work than mere gum lines, tooth fairies and molar size. How the jaw is shaped, when it develops and even how "normally" it develops can all affect the placement, even the comfort, of your child's teeth.

When the upper and lower teeth grow at different rates, or times, or even when the lower jaw grows disproportionately with the upper jaw, something known as a "crossbite" can occur.

Your child might have a crossbite if, for instance, the lower jaw is out of line with the upper jaw (kind of like a box that won't close right because one of the hinges is bent).

Or perhaps on the right side of your child's mouth, the lower teeth "stick out" a little farther than the top teeth, making the upper teeth on his right side overlap in turn.

Or, maybe, your child's upper and lower jaws are out of alignment so that instead of the top and bottom front teeth meeting "naturally" as they should, the front teeth fall somewhat behind the lower teeth. This would be the reverse of an overbite.

As you might imagine, any or all of these developments can lead to short- and long-term discomfort for your child.

How, When & Why Crossbites Form

You might be amazed to find out how many ways a crossbite can form as your child grows and develops during his or her formative years. Heredity is one key to jaw growth, or alignment, as is the size – big or small – of your child's developing jaw.

Another factor that can contribute to the development of a potential crossbite is if it takes your child too long to lose his or her baby teeth. In some extreme cases, in fact, if it takes too long for your child to lose his baby teeth, another set of teeth can grow in behind them, throwing the alignment off and contributing to a crossbite.

Believe it or not, something as basic as whether your child breathes through her nose or her mouth can also contribute to a crossbite. While most children breathe through their noses, some children develop a habit early on of breathing through their mouths instead.

In children who breathe through their noses while they're sleeping, the tongue naturally rests on the roof of the mouth, promoting natural and proper upper jaw growth.

When young children breathe through their mouths, however, the tongue "relocates" from the roof of the mouth to the bottom, removing that extra support and potentially contributing to reduced upper jaw bone growth; this can create the "crossbite" we spoke of previously.

How Can I Spot a Crossbite?

Although it sounds severe – and even painful – from the description provided above, the effects of a crossbite can take time to manifest themselves. Still, here are some of the tell tale signs that your child might be cultivating, or already suffering from, a crossbite:

- **Snoring**
- **Difficulty breathing**
- **Chewing on one side of the mouth or the other**
- **Signs of an under bite, or the upper teeth coming to rest behind the lower teeth**
- **Painful chewing**

- **If your child's chin seems "off center" or disproportionate**

- o Etc.

How, When & Why to Correct a Crossbite

Where should you start to look for treatment if you're concerned about your child's jaw development after reading this section? If you suspect your child might have a crossbite, approach your family dentist about a recommendation for a specialist such as an orthodontist.

There are many possible treatments available for a crossbite, and your orthodontist can work with you closely to make the right and specific decisions for you and your child.

When should you start? I believe you know my standard answer when it comes to questions like this one: **as early as possible**! The same way that an auto mechanic would tell you to take care of that oil leak, bulging tire or faulty timing belt sooner rather than later, myself and my colleagues in orthodontics will always favor early treatment to later.

The fact is that crossbites are often closely linked with other orthodontic issues, such as teeth alignment, jaw size and growth. Naturally, the sooner you address any or all of these issues, the better.

Finally, why should you address a crossbite? Crossbites can lead to pain, discomfort and lack of confidence as your child begins to feel insecure or even ostracized because of this very treatable, very normal series of jaw and teeth developments.

Not only can crossbites become physically uncomfortable if left untreated, but if the misalignment or root cause of the bite isn't fixed in early childhood, then the child's appearance and, ultimately, confidence could be affected as the crossbite becomes more pronounced in adolescence.

Question # 12:
Do They Still Make Metal Braces?

The fact is, metal braces still have a valued place in the orthodontic world, and despite advances and breakthroughs of products like Invisalign and even clear braces, aren't going extinct anytime soon!

Why are metal braces still so popular? Well, for one thing, metal braces are very strong and can withstand most types of treatment. Today's metal braces are smaller, sleeker, and more polished than ever before.

Older, traditional metal braces require an elastic o-shaped rubber band, called a ligature to hold the arch wire onto the bracket. These elastic ties collect more plaque and bacteria, making it harder for patients to clean the teeth and gums.

You may have heard of "speed braces." These are sometimes also referred to as "self-ligating brackets" or "tie-free braces." Self-ligating means that the brackets do not need the little o-shaped rubber bands (ligatures) or metal tie wires to hold the arch wire onto the bracket. Several companies have developed braces for holding the wires in place without ligatures.

By using self-ligation technology, the brackets allow the wire to slide back and forth. This advancement allows for fewer adjustments and fewer appointments. These types of braces do not need rubber bands to hold the arch wire in place. They use a "door" to secure the arch wire to the bracket. They are smaller than traditional metal and less food gets trapped around them when you eat.

Your orthodontist might use an advanced self-ligating bracket that does not require physical tightening of the wire to the braces. It is a twin bracket made of metal or clear ceramic, and utilizes a special built-in clip. The pressure from specific types of arch wires activates the clip and delivers specific amounts of force to each tooth, resulting in fast, directed results.

Naturally, orthodontists are very excited about the hygiene benefits of these self-closing or tie-free metal braces. Patients are excited that their braces are small, smooth, friction-free and straighten their teeth in fewer visits with less discomfort than braces with wires that are "tied-in."

Question # 13:
What's the Deal with Clear Braces?

Ceramic braces are very strong and generally do not stain. Two popular brands are Clarity, made by 3M Unitek; and In-Ovation C, made by GAC. Adults like to choose ceramic because they "blend in" with the teeth and are less noticeable than metal. These are the type of braces actor Tom Cruise had.

Older types of ceramic braces required white or clear ligatures (tiny rubber bands) to hold the wire on to the braces. In-Ovation C is a revolutionary tie-free ceramic braces system that combines the same efficient tooth movement with exceptional esthetics. Patients choosing In-Ovation C no longer have to decide between metal braces or clear braces that could stain.

Today's clear In-Ovation C braces are very esthetic because they no longer require the small rubber bands that could stain with certain foods or drinks.

Adult Orthodontics

It's not uncommon for individuals who have undergone orthodontic treatment earlier in life to find their teeth have drifted out of alignment over the years. Most adults won't think twice about bleaching their teeth to roll back the effects of time. Yet few think about the role orthodontics can play.

Adults of all ages can enjoy the same cosmetic and health benefits of properly aligned teeth with In-Ovation C system braces.

"My friends often complain about having a 'metal smile' but with In-Ovation C, you can hardly notice you are wearing braces. I see an improvement in my smile and I am really glad I have In-Ovation C braces."

~ Haley

Benefits Beyond Beauty

Improperly aligned teeth can do more than undermine your confidence. They can make proper cleaning and brushing more difficult, contribute to enamel loss and even set the stage for more significant problems down the road. Fortunately, discrete treatment with In-Ovation C braces can help keep you aligned with a healthy, happy lifestyle.

The Solution is Clear

Orthodontists believe that every individual has the right to live their life with a smile they truly love, particularly children. Healthy, straight, attractive smiles don't just make your child healthier but happier and more self-confidence. And isn't that what we all want for them?

In-Ovation C helps you achieve the smile of your dreams faster, easier and more discretely than you ever imagined. Embrace the confidence that comes with beautifully aligned teeth and put your smile on display. Schedule a consultation and ask your orthodontist if In-Ovation C system braces are right for you.

Faster Treatment; Fewer Appointments

The In-Ovation C system use a free-sliding technology that places almost no pressure on your teeth as it gently corrects their alignment. Less pressure means a more comfortable treatment.

With In-Ovation C free-sliding braces, your treatment can proceed faster with fewer follow up visits than traditional fixed wire braces.

Question # 14:
What is Invisalign?

No doubt you've heard all about the revolutionary Invisalign® system for teeth straightening. Chances are, though, that while you're familiar with the brand name of this amazing new product, you might not be familiar with exactly how the system works. In this section I'll answer the most frequently asked questions about Invisalign.

For starters, the Invisalign system is the virtually invisible way to straighten your teeth and achieve the dazzling smile you've always dreamed of. Using advanced 3-D computer-imaging technology, Invisalign depicts your complete treatment plan, from the initial position of your teeth to the final desired position.

After that, a series of clear aligners are custom-made for your teeth – and your teeth only – to move them little by little. Each aligner is worn for about two weeks before being replaced by the next in the series, until the final position of your teeth is achieved. When will that be, exactly? The amount and duration of each aligner series differs for every mouth. Your Invisalign treatment time will be determined by your doctor, based on your specific needs.

What are the primary benefits of Invisalign?

Like the word that inspired them, Invisalign aligners are practically clear; or as close to "invisible" as one can get. No one may even notice that you're wearing these virtually invisible "braces," making Invisalign a seamless fit with your lifestyle and day-to-day interactions with others.

Invisalign is also removable. Unlike braces, you have the flexibility to eat and drink whatever you want during treatment by simply removing the aligners before a meal or snack. And you can also remove the aligners to brush and floss as you normally would for fresh breath and good oral hygiene.

Unlike braces, there are no metal brackets or wires that could cause irritation to your mouth with the Invisalign system. Furthermore, since your office visits during treatment don't involve metal or wire adjustments, you will likely spend less time in the doctor's chair (and that's always a good thing for young patients!).

Finally, Invisalign allows you to view your virtual results and treatment plan before you start so you can see how your straight teeth will look when your treatment is complete.

How do I get started with Invisalign?

It's simple: just make an appointment with your local orthodontist for an initial consultation. Most doctors will offer a free initial consultation to see if you are a good candidate for Invisalign.

If yours doesn't, consider finding an orthodontist who does!

How will Invisalign effectively move my teeth?

Aligners are the foundation for, and work in concert with, the Invisalign system. Like brackets and arch wires are to braces, Invisalign aligners move teeth through the appropriate placement of controlled force on your child's teeth. The main difference is that Invisalign not only controls forces, but also the timing of the force application.

During each stage, only certain teeth are allowed to move. These movements are determined by your doctor as he or she maps out your unique Invisalign treatment plan.

What are aligners made of, and what do they look like?

The virtually invisible aligners, which are made of a thermoplastic material uniquely developed for the Invisalign treatment plan, look similar to tooth-whitening trays. Invisalign aligners are custom-made for you and only you to move your teeth in the sequence determined by your doctor.

How old is the technology?

In 1945, Dr. H.D. Kesling envisioned that one day modern technology would enable the use of a series of tooth positioners to produce the kinds of movements required for comprehensive orthodontic treatment.

Technology has made this vision a reality. Using advanced computer technology, Align Technology produces Invisalign, a series of customized clear appliances, or aligners. Each aligner is worn sequentially by the patient to produce extensive tooth movements in both upper and lower arches.

How many patients are being treated with Invisalign?

More than 1,000,000 patients worldwide have been treated with Invisalign. The number of Invisalign smiles grows daily. Will your child's be next?!?

Has the FDA cleared Invisalign?

Invisalign aligners are classified as Class II medical devices by the FDA, and Align Technology, Inc. has held the necessary 510K clearance from the FDA since 1998 to be able to sell and market the Invisalign system.

Do Invisalign aligners contain Bisphenol-A (BPA)?

No. Invisalign aligners and Vivera Retainers do not contain Bisphenol-A or phthalate plasticizers. These aligners and retainers are made with USP Class VI medical grade, high molecular weight, polyurethane resins.

Tests have been conducted to determine the biocompatibility of these materials, and show that they are biocompatible and pass all applicable regulatory requirements and thresholds for human wear in the mouth. Of course, as with any medical device, you should consult with your health professional about your aligner or retainer treatment and any applicable risks of use.

Question # 15:
What's So Special About Invisalign Teen?

You no longer have to straighten your teeth the old-fashioned way, with metal braces. Much like its more "grown up" version, the Invisalign Teen System lets you do it the modern, hygienic way. Your new smile is created with the most innovative technology – a series of clear aligners that are custom-fit to your teeth.

The first thing you should know is that an average treatment takes about a year. Plus your treatment can begin even if you don't have all of your permanent teeth. Invisalign Teen was designed to meet your needs. Let's find out more about this revolutionary new system and to see if it's right for you and your child.

How does Invisalign Teen work?

Aligners snap on your teeth easily. They are comfortable and practically invisible. Invisalign Teen allows for your growing permanent teeth and gently and continuously moves your teeth in small increments. Aligners are worn for about two weeks, then you swap them for a new pair.

Invisalign Teen aligners have a Blue Dot Wear Indicator, designed to show an estimation of wear-time. The dot is designed to fade until it's clear over a two-week period if you wear your aligners properly (meaning for 20 to 22 hours every day).

The Benefits of Invisalign Teen

Invisalign Teen™ is designed to custom-fit your teeth and go with your lifestyle. During your treatment, you can keep smiling, playing sports, eating what you want, and brushing and flossing normally.

Plus, unlike traditional braces, the aligners are made of smooth plastic and move your teeth gradually.

Your aligners can be removed for eating, brushing, and flossing, or going to a special event. The aligners are replaceable if lost. That's right; you get up to six free individual aligners.

After your Invisalign Teen treatment, you may find your self-confidence boosted by your new smile and the change in your appearance. Some people even feel that way during treatment. As you know, smiling has many benefits. It can help you make a strong impression in lots of different social situations – at school, at work, or at a party.

Treatable Conditions

Invisalign Teen really works. It helps correct a broad range of dental and orthodontic issues. You can get a confident smile without metal bands, brackets, or wires.

It works on many kinds of conditions, including: overly crowded teeth, widely spaced teeth, crossbites, overbites, and under bites.

Question # 16:
What in the Heck is Incognito by 3M?

Brought to you by the brilliant minds at 3M, you are about to discover a completely different way to wear braces. Incognito is the only fully-customizable lingual (inside of your teeth) braces system on the market.

To help me explain the majesty and wonder that is this revolutionary new system, I've comprised what I call The 3 I's of Incognito:

The First "I" of Incognito: *Invisible*

iBraces (now known as Incognito) Orthodontic Braces are a new generation of orthodontic braces for teens and adults. Because they are placed behind your teeth, no one will ever know you are wearing braces unless you tell them. The Incognito Appliances can give you a beautiful smile, even while you're wearing them.

The Second "I" of Incognito: *Individualized*

Incognito Appliances are the only 100% customized fixed appliance system for invisible orthodontic treatment on the U.S. market today. They are created using state-of-the-art technology and are completely customized to the shape of your teeth and to your dental situation. And they have the unique prescription that your orthodontist creates for you built-in, to ensure you get the results that you want.

The Third "I" of Incognito: *Intelligent*

With the Incognito System you get efficient, effective tooth movement and great aesthetics. From the outset, the brackets and wires are engineered to deliver targeted results.

PART 4

Financing the Whole Thing Without Breaking the Bank

Question # 17:
How Do I Pay for My New Smile?

Like any major dental or even medical procedure, orthodontic procedures can cost several thousand dollars, not all of which is covered by your insurance (depending on the plan; see below).

How much you may have to pay out of pocket depends on the type of procedure and, of course, the specifics of your insurance policy. One way many of my patients pay for their procedures is by utilizing the benefits of what is known as "Flex Spending," where an account through their work can be used to pay for braces with pre-tax dollars.

Three Ways to Eliminate Flex Spending Headaches (Almost) Instantly

How can you make the most of your employer's Flex Plan so that the amount out of your pocket is reduced to a more manageable figure? Here are three solutions you can take action on starting today:

The First Way: *Sign Up Early*

Preparation is key to success in any endeavor. So to make the most of your Flex Plan, **set aside your flex spending dollars now**. Many employers set higher limits than you think on the amount of Flex Spending Dollars you can contribute each year, tax-free, from your salary to pay for health care expenses like orthodontic treatment.

Case in point: Many employers allow $2,500 or even $5,000 of pre-tax earnings to be set aside for your flex plan. Are you getting all of that money you can to pay for your child's orthodontic care?

Maybe; maybe not. Failing to sign up early could cost you more in out-of-pocket orthodontic expenses, especially if your plan is not set up and ready before your child's orthodontic treatment begins. If you have a new plan, work with your plan administrator to sign up early for next year in order to maximize your savings!

The Second Way: *Make Your Employer Aware of Family Status Change*

Different employers have different sign-up deadlines for the Flex plans, but typically at the beginning of the year, your employer asks you how much money you want to contribute to your Flex Plan for the year.

The problem with making annual decisions about your healthcare coverage is that you only have one opportunity to enroll, unless you have a qualified "family status change."

So what, exactly, IS a "family status" change? Family Status changes like marriage, birth, divorce or loss of a spouse's insurance coverage are qualified reasons to change your plan, and possibly add more coverage for orthodontic treatment.

The Third Way: *Choose Wisely!*

Finally, give some thought to calculating how much money to contribute to your flex plan at work this year. If you are considering orthodontic treatment, visit your doctor's office for an initial consultation.

Your treatment coordinator(s) can help you plan exactly how much money you should contribute to help reduce your out-of-pocket expenses when it's time to actually pay for, and receive, the procedure.

Here's something you may not know about your friendly flex plan: If you put in more money than you need, by law, you lose the money! You have three months after the end of the calendar year to submit claims for eligible expenses from the previous calendar year. Any money left in your account after this three month period is lost.

Question # 18:
Does My Insurance Cover the Cost of Braces?

These days there are as many different types of insurance plans as there are patients in my office. I can't possibly speak to your unique and personal insurance policy without seeing it first but, in general, my experience tells me that "most" insurance policies cover "some" of your orthodontic expenses.

I realize that answer sounds very vague but here are a couple of variables you need to answer before an insurance agent can help you determine what, how long and how many procedures fall under your insurance:

- **The type of procedure (braces, Invisalign, etc.)**
- **The duration of the procedure (two months, six months, a year, etc.)**
- **The cause of the procedure (a patient presenting with pain, a parent's concern, traumatic injury or accident, congenital birth defect like cleft lip or palate etc.)**
- **The nature of the procedure (to correct pain/discomfort, cosmetic, etc.)**
- **Etc.**

My point is, this one question I can only partially answer, but here is one thing I'm certain of: talking to your insurance agent will help you get the right answers you need.

TIP : keep an insurance journal of every interaction with your carrier. Write down the date, time of call, name of the person you contacted, and the exact instructions or recommendations following the call. Later, if your insurance company doesn't remember what they told you, you'll have it accurately written down. If they still don't remember, ask them to pull the recorded audio tape from your previous call, so that you can accurately "remind" them of exactly what they told you.

Question # 19:
How Can I Really Save a Bundle on Braces?

Here are eighteen controversial ways to save some *real* money when paying for your child's braces. Why are they controversial? Well, I say they are controversial because most orthodontists don't want to think about unique ways to save you money. Why? Because the more money you save, the less they make; period.

However, I'm a firm believer in giving everyone the opportunity to get a great smile if they *really* want one. Finances shouldn't stand in the way of a safe, healthy and comfortable smile. After all, your child's confidence depends on it!

So here are eighteen fast, simple and effective ways to get creative. Along the way, you might just be surprised the amount of savings you can find.

1. **Get braces in April or November and see if you can save a little extra by paying in full.** These are the months that orthodontists are the least-busy, and it's when we have our most meetings (April-May). In November everyone is getting ready for the holidays or the office is closed the week of Thanksgiving. By scheduling during the "off season," you can often find better deals with willing orthodontists.

2. **See if you can get a discount for not breaking any brackets.** Believe it or not, most orthodontists would happily take $100 off your final bill if you don't break any appliances throughout treatment!

3. **New technology; better pricing.** See if you can be one of your orthodontist's first patients with a new technology and

save some money on the lab fee or receive a discount for being a teaching case.

4. **See if your local dental school has an orthodontic program.** The treatment at such institutions is supervised by board-certified orthodontists (most of whom practice in the surrounding area). While you might spend a little more time in the chair as a teaching case, if you have the time, it might be well worth the wait because you can save up to **half the cost of traditional braces**.

5. **Ask your insurance plans when they send out their fee schedules to participating providers.** If the insurance company updates their fees or the orthodontist raises his or her fees to keep up with the cost of inflation, it might be around November in preparation for the next year.

6. **See your dentist every 4-6 months.** While you're wearing your braces, the extra cleaning each year can prevent tooth decay, a costly item to repair.

7. **Get your flex spending dollars in order with your employer.** If you set money aside in a Flex Plan, it may be "tax-free" but it comes with some stipulations: namely, you have to use it before the end of the year – or else you lose it.

8. **See if you can get a second set of retainers from your orthodontist at the end of treatment.** Sometimes getting two sets of retainers at the same time can be cheaper than buying a second set later in life when you lose or break your first set.

9. **See if your husband or wife has an insurance plan that covers braces.** Be sure to enroll in the plan with enough time to spare before your child needs braces, so that the procedure is not denied by your insurance company due to a waiting period.

10. **Ask for flexible financing options.** When you boil it down to the basics, your orthodontist really just wants to help you. Regardless of his specialty, your doctor spent way too much time in school NOT to love what he does. What's more, if you're easy to work with, keep your teeth clean and avoid breaking your braces while you're wearing them, he or she will probably be thrilled to help you finance the care – or find another way to afford the investment.

11. **Do you have multiple kids in treatment?** If so, take advantage of that fact and see if you can get a "family discount."

12. **If finances are extremely tight, you should check out the organizations that orthodontists have created to help provide pro-bono care, such as SmilesChangeLives.org.** There are even more foundations like this if you have a cleft palate or other facial anomalies, like the Rheam Foundation for Cleft and Craniofacial Research.

13. **School Auctions, Churches or public service entities will often receive donations from local orthodontists wishing to donate a case to the school or organization for a fundraiser.** Checking around the local school newsletters or Church bulletin for their upcoming silent auctions could be a great find! If you're not willing to leave such things to chance, call your local schools or churches and ask them

specifically if they have such a fund and, if so, how to apply/qualify.

14. **If you're thinking about a career change, apply at your local orthodontist's office.** Most orthodontists offer free braces to their staff and their children as an employee benefit! (And you never know, you could love your career AND your child's new braces!)

15. **Military, school teacher and fire fighters sometimes receive special courtesies in dental and orthodontic offices throughout the year.** Keep your ear to the ground and you might save a few bucks or at least get a donation from the orthodontist to your organization.

16. **This tactic won't save you any money, but it could earn your organization or business some money if you have a newsletter, sports team, fund raiser or special event that needs a sponsor.** Ask your orthodontist. Most orthodontic offices are huge supporters of the communities in which they practice and would probably love to advertise with your organization.

17. **Got taxes?** Good! Why not use your tax refund to help pay for treatment in full and ask for a courtesy on the average fees associated with financing a full orthodontic case. In some areas, you can save as much as 10% on the cost of braces by simply saving your pennies and paying the entire bill at once, up front.

18. **Ask for more-flexible financing, either through a third party credit company like Chase Healthcare Advance, CareCredit or in-house financing through your**

orthodontist. Most orthodontists will accept a reasonable down-payment and split the remaining amount into easy monthly payments for your convenience. With automated withdrawals from a checking or savings account, you might be able to stretch the monthly payments out over a longer period to make each payment lower. Just don't be shocked if your orthodontist asks you to approve a credit check. A little homework up front can be well worth the effort when your monthly orthodontic bill is lower than your cable TV bill!

There's no doubt about it; braces can be expensive. However, now that you're armed with these eighteen massive, budget-saving tips, you won't need to decide between braces and your budget ever again!

PART 5

Following Good Advice for Fantastic Results

Question # 20:
How Should My Child Brush with Braces?

Now that your child has braces on for the duration (however long, or short, that duration might be), you must make sure your child brushes his or her teeth and gums better than ever before.

Extra care must be taken in the area between the gums and your child's appliance. Food that collects around the braces and wires can cause swollen gums, permanent stains (decalcification or white spots), and cavities.

Here are some simple tips you can share with your child for the best results when brushing with braces on:

- **Brush your teeth with a medium nylon toothbrush after you eat and before bed.**
- **Brush, rinse, and look; if you find any areas that are not clean, brush them again.**
- **Brush your gums as you brush your teeth (massage and stimulate).**
- **If no toothpaste is available, brush without.**
- **If you are unable to brush, rinse your mouth vigorously with water.**
- **Replace your old toothbrush when it gets worn out.**
- **It is absolutely essential that you continue regular visits to your family dentist for checkups and cleanings throughout your orthodontic treatment!**

Question # 21:
Are There Any Foods My Child Should Avoid With Braces?

After your child's orthodontic appliance has been placed, the teeth will be tender to biting pressure for 5 to 10 days. This is absolutely normal. Of course, this can vary with different patients so be sure to monitor your child's discomfort level carefully.

During this period of tenderness, softer foods are recommended for your child, such as soups, macaroni, spaghetti, fish, eggs, yogurt, Jello, milkshakes, etc. Tylenol® or Advil® will help relieve any discomfort. Warm salt-water rinses are also helpful (see earlier tip for specific directions). Use the soft white wax provided by your orthodontist where it is needed.

Continue to monitor what foods your child eats. Hard and sticky foods will break off brackets, bend wires, and loosen bands, which will extend your child's total treatment time. Foods high in sugar can cause cavities, calculus build-up, and ugly stains on your child's teeth.

So, what can you do, as a parent, to make the most of the time while your child has his or her braces on? You must limit your child's diet to softer, healthy foods. There are certain types of foods that must be avoided during orthodontic treatment:

- Hard Foods: Ice, nuts, popcorn, peanut brittle, rock candy, apples & carrots (unless cut into pieces), corn on the cob, hard pretzels, hard rolls, bagels, hard tacos, corn chips.
- Sticky Foods: Jolly Ranchers, caramels, bubble gum, taffy, suckers, Starburst candy, Dots / jelly candies.
- Chewy Foods: Pizza crust, crusty breads, beef jerky, gummy bears; avoid chewing on pens and pencils.

- Sugary Foods and Drinks: This would include things like cake, ice cream, cookies, pie, candy, soda pop, drinks with sugar.

Question # 22:
What Should I Do in Case of an Orthodontic Emergency or Injury?

While orthodontists recognize that most "emergencies" having to do with braces are not life-and-death situations, we also understand that situations may occur that cause discomfort and even pain.

Perhaps a wire breaks or you accidentally eat something that causes a problem, such as sticky taffy or a burger bun with sesame seeds. I have provided the information below to help you prevent those types of emergencies and also to answer some of the most common questions regarding these special situations.

If you are experiencing an orthodontic emergency that can't wait for regular office hours, most orthodontic offices have a special number to call, either before, during or after business hours. If this information isn't given to you readily, check to see how your doctor's office handles emergencies. Remember, information is power and the time to ask about a 24-hour emergency call center number is before your child loses a bracket or eats a piece of toffee, not after!

When Emergencies (Really) Aren't!

Some emergencies actually aren't. Or, if they are, can be easily and safely remedied at home. Case in point: teeth, when moving, can be really tender for about a week after the initial placement of the orthodontic appliances and also after each adjustment.

Discomfort can be relieved by over-the-counter pain relievers such as Tylenol or Motrin. Follow the dosage recommendations and any additional precautions as listed on the bottle. Some patients find it helpful to take the first dose at the appointment time to help prevent some of the discomfort to come when the teeth start to move.

During the first two weeks, the inside of your cheeks will be tender because they are not used to the braces. As time goes by, the inside of the cheeks will toughen up and adjust to the braces. While the cheeks are still sensitive, using wax on the rough spots can be very helpful. Also helpful are warm saltwater rinses which soothe the cheek lining (see instructions below).

Some inconveniences while going through treatment are normal. Many times repairs can be put off until your next regular appointment. Of course, your orthodontist is there to serve you and encourage you to call any time you have a question.

Special Feature: *Making a Saltwater Rinse*

To make a salt water rinse, mix ½ teaspoon of table salt in one cup of warm water. Stir until the salt is completely dissolved. Gently swish about ¼ of the cup in your mouth for 30 seconds. Make sure you force the water over the areas that feel sore. Then spit the water into the sink. Repeat until the entire cup is gone.

Question # 23: *Where Can I Find the Best Athletic Mouth Guard for My Child's Braces?*

Since the time that most kids wear braces typically also falls into the time when most kids are the most active, the issue of "sports versus braces" often comes up in my orthodontist's office.

The fact is, the two shouldn't be mutually exclusive. Now more than ever, modern technology and the rise in affordable, quality sports equipment should mean that no child should have to choose between sports and straight teeth!

Often, the issue boils down to finding a proper mouth guard, not only for the sport in question but the child in question. Naturally, as a concerned parent, you will want only the best for your child.

But... where to start?

Purchasing the "best" mouth guard can be a frustrating task for athletes and parents alike. Fortunately, multiple options exist. Custom mouth guards and off-the-shelf varieties can both be effective if **worn properly** and selected for the **appropriate level of play**.

In a recent review article in *Clinics in Sports Medicine*, Dr. Daneshvar and colleagues in the Department of Neurology at Boston University School of Medicine examined what the literature says about different types of mouth guards and the rate of sports-related concussions.

To date, there have been "no large studies published in the scientific community that can demonstrate a significant difference in the type of mouth guard used and the rate of concussions."

When used properly, mouth guards can provide "an additional level of protection against dental injuries." Many popular mouth guards offer free insurance for financial protection in the event of a dental injury. One might consider this option if there is a concern of future dental treatment or a history of chipped teeth related to sports injuries.

The best advice for patients or parents looking for a mouth guard can be obtained from your pediatrician, dentist, pediatric dentist, orthodontist or oral surgeon. All of these specialists are uniquely trained to offer customized advice in order to help you prevent a sports-related dental or facial injury.

References: Daneshvar DH, Baugh CM, Nowinski CJ, McKee AC, Stern RA, Cantu RC. Helmets and mouth guards : the role of personal equipment in preventing sport-related concussions. Clin Sports Med. 2011 Jan; 30(1) : 145-63.

Question # 24:
Why Are Retainers So Important?

So, your child's braces are off and they're ready to live a life of confidence and good oral health. Well, yes and no; the fact is, once the braces come off, there is still just a little more work to do.

How much work? It depends; I like to think of wearing your braces as only half of the teeth-straightening solution. What's the second half? Retainers!

While many of my patients are eager to be done with braces once they come off, the fact is that retainers do as much work – if not more – than the braces themselves. Straight teeth don't just get that way; they stay that way – and retainers help.

Why are retainers so important? Once your child's braces come off you want the teeth to stay in position. After all, they've worked so hard for so many months to achieve straight, healthy teeth – why stumble at the finish line?

That's what can happen if your child forgets to or, more likely, simply chooses not to wear his or her retainer. While the braces come off, the teeth can still shift if not allowed a period of adjustment to settle in. The retainer gives this "adjustment period" by gently but purposefully keeping your child's straight teeth straight!

Years ago, patients and clinicians alike thought you could straighten your teeth and they would stay straight forever. However, research has now shown that the only way to guarantee straight teeth for life is through the use of fixed or removable retainers for life.[1]

As we age, teeth naturally shift to the middle and crowd. Combined with late growth of the lower jaw, shifting of the teeth is expected following orthodontic treatment.[2]

Therefore, retainers are extremely important in the maintenance of your new smile following orthodontic treatment. This chapter describes why retainers are so important and how your child can use them properly to ensure straight teeth for a lifetime.

Factors Affecting Treatment Stability

Many of our patients ask what type of retainer we recommend. "Can I get a clear retainer?" or "Will I need a fixed retainer?" are common patient questions. Your orthodontist takes into account several factors when he or she plans to retain the positions of your teeth.

Growth of the jaws following treatment, the amount of time needed for gum and bone tissues to stabilize, and pressures from the lips and tongue are all important factors that affect the stability of your finished result.[3] After considering these factors, your orthodontist decides what type of retainer you should wear and how long you should wear it.

Fixed Retainer

A fixed retainer is typically placed (glued) on the inside surfaces of the lower front teeth. This type of retainer can be attached to the two canine teeth or to every tooth in the area. A fixed retainer is very efficient at maintaining the positions of the teeth in certain situations.[4] If your orthodontist decides to place a fixed retainer, it will make cleaning between your teeth more difficult.

Ask your orthodontist, dentist, and dental hygienist for tips and tricks to help you keep your teeth clean while wearing a fixed retainer. With proper care and regular visits to your general dentist, your fixed retainer can be left in place until lower jaw growth is completed (early adulthood) or indefinitely, as indicated.[3]

Removable Retainers

When your child thinks of a retainer, chances are he or she is picturing a "removable retainer." That's because removable retainers have been used successfully for many years and are probably the most common type of retainer. Patients identify immediately with the wire that runs across the front teeth to help maintain tooth alignment and symmetry.

The Hawley retainer is probably the most popular type of removable retainer. It is made of plastic and stainless steel wire and is custom-made for your mouth and teeth. Variations of this type of retainer are too numerous to list, but they all achieve the same result – maintenance of your new smile for life.

Since removable retainers can be taken out, patients frequently ask how long they need to wear the retainer. Most relapse, or unwanted tooth movement, occurs in the first 3-6 months after the braces are removed.

For the average patient, your child will wear his or her removable retainer full-time for the first 3-6 months, and thereafter only while sleeping. If your child's orthodontist recommends a period of time longer or shorter than this, don't be alarmed; he or she is only protecting your child's smile against the factors we mentioned at the beginning of the article.

For example, a patient with severely misaligned jaws and teeth might wear retainers for a longer duration than a patient with only minor tooth-alignment problems. If you are unsure of his or her retention program, be sure to ask your child's orthodontist or orthodontic assistant for specific instructions regarding the wear and care of your child's retainers.

Clear or Invisible Retainers

With the advent of new, clear plastic materials in orthodontics, patients can benefit from more esthetic options during the retention phase of orthodontic treatment. Clear retainers are comfortable, esthetic, and require no adjustment. However, they can be severely worn or broken if subjected to heavy biting forces.

In our office, patients receive clear retainers as a back-up retainer and for social convenience during the first 3-6 months. If the Hawley retainer is lost or broken, the clear retainer can be used as a back-up, while our lab fabricates a new Hawley retainer. We have found this program to be very beneficial in maintaining healthy, beautiful smiles for life.

Retainers – What to Expect

Hearing that your child may need to wear a retainer may seem like a scary thing at first. But that's probably because you are not familiar with what they are and what they do. Once we help you take the mystery out of retainers for you and your child, it will be clear to see that they are a simple device that helps to correct your child's bite, as well as sometimes address other conditions.

And, we promise, they are nothing to be afraid of!

What They Are

You may have seen people wearing a retainer before, but they are not all that noticeable. A retainer is a small device that is made out of clear plastic, rubber, or even metal. They are custom-made so that they only fit your teeth. They are part of a treatment plan that has likely been determined by an orthodontist.

Using retainers to help align teeth is a common option. The length of time that someone has to wear them varies, but they are especially common following someone having their braces removed. During the process of wearing braces, the teeth have been moved into the desired position, but they are not yet settled into the gum and jaw.

By using a retainer, it helps to further set your child's teeth in their new position. Teeth tend to shift, so the retainer can help keep them where they are supposed to be until they are settled in and will not shift out of place.

Reasons for Wearing

Wearing a retainer after having braces removed is just one of the ways retainers are used. During this route, the retainer is typically worn each day for a period of six months, then your child will wear it to bed at night for a while. This effort just helps to ensure that the new tooth placement is retained.

There are other conditions that call for a retainer as part of corrective treatment as well. Some of those conditions include:

To close any gaps that may be in the bite.
To help correct speech problems or
A variety of medical conditions, including tongue thrust, where the tongue goes between the teeth when talking.
Retainers can also be used to address bruxism, which is the grinding of the teeth while sleeping.

There are a variety of conditions that may call for a treatment plan that requires a retainer. Working with an orthodontist is the best way to determine if one can help with a particular condition and how long one would have to be worn, as the time varies depending on the severity of the problem being treated.

Preparing for a Retainer

When a retainer is being recommended as part of your child's treatment plan, it helps to know what to expect, such as a mold being made of your child's teeth. This is done through a process of using a thick liquid, called alginate, which makes a temporary mold of the teeth. That temporary mold is then used to make the retainer.

Retainers today have come a long way from the bigger pure metal ones of decades past. They can be customized to show your child's personality, including having colors and pictures on them, or they can be clear plastic so that they are less noticeable to others. Depending on who is getting the retainer and their age, there are many options to consider.

Length, Care and Beyond

The length of time your child can expect to wear his or her retainer varies. Much of that variety will depend on the reason and severity of the treatment he or she is receiving. Your child can expect to meet with the orthodontist periodically, in order to make sure that everything is going according to the treatment plan and there is no discomfort.

Caring for a retainer is simple because they can easily be removed. It is recommended that they are cleaned daily, in order to maintain good oral hygiene and get rid of plaque and food particles. How the retainer is cleaned depends upon the type that your child has, so you will need to check with the orthodontist for the cleaning recommendations on your specific version.

Retainers are part of a treatment plan that may be addressing the misalignment of the teeth, close gaps in the bite, correct speech problems, and even assist in medical conditions.

Retainers are a simple device that can do an important job. Whether helping to get teeth settled in after braces, to align teeth, or to correct another condition, they are a treatment option that helps people to feel confident, as well as more comfortable.

While they may seem like a "nuisance" after your child has spent so long in braces, why risk letting all the hard work he or she has already done go down the tubes when a simple appliance can help ensure straight teeth for life?

References:

1. Little RM, Riedel RA, Artun J. An evaluation of changes in mandibular anterior alignment from 10 to 20 years postretention. American Journal of Orthodontics and Dentofacial Orthopedics; 1988 (93): 423-428.
2. Nanda RS, Nanda SK. Considerations of dentofacial growth in long-term retention and stability : is active retention needed? American Journal of Orthodontics and Dentofacial Orthopedics. 1992 (101): 297-302.
3. English JD, Peltomäki T, Pham-Litschel K. Mosby's Orthodontic Review. St. Louis : Mosby, 2009, pp 265-270.
4. Espen HD, Zachrisson BU. Long-term experience with direct bonded lingual retainers. Journal of Clinical Orthodontics; 1991 (10): 619-630.

Bonus Chapter:
7 Ways to Celebrate Getting Your Braces Off!

Having braces on your teeth can last from a few months to a few years, depending upon all the factors involved. And during the time that you have had them on your teeth, you probably felt like you missed out on a lot! There are things you couldn't eat at all, things you had to cut up real small, and most likely you longed for the day that you could sink your teeth into an apple!

Time to Celebrate

So the day is finally in sight. It's time to get the braces off and give your teeth and mouth the freedom for which you have been waiting. Now is the time to celebrate!

There are so many ways that you can celebrate, everything from writing a journal about your experience to recording a video that shares your experience and shows your new look.

Here are seven options that you may want to consider:

- **Throw a party**. Throwing a braces are off party is a great way to celebrate. Invite your friends over, put out the Doritos that you have been longing for, and enjoy showing off those new straight teeth. Your friends will love being able to take part in your celebration.
- **Plan a photo shoot**. You deserve to show the world your new beautiful smile! Plan a photo shoot, so you can be one-on-one with a photographer and put your best smile forward. You will get some great shots and can show all your MySpace or

Facebook friends your new look. You may even want to complete the whole look by making your photo shoot one of the glamour shot ones, where you get the make-up and hair pampering right before the shoot.

- **Chew some gum**. You know you have been wanting to have gum for the longest time. Although it's not a good thing to still do regularly, you can take an afternoon to chew some gum and feel guilt and worry free. Chew to your heart's content!
- **Go caramel**. Now is the time that you can sink your teeth into a caramel apple. No more avoiding the caramel and cutting the apple into bite-sized pieces. Nope, you can actually eat a full caramel apple, right off the stick! Get one at the mall, a carnival, or have fun making them yourself. Either way, you will love being able to bite into that sticky gooey sweetness worry free!
- **Picnic in the park**. Weather permitting, a picnic in the park will make for a fun celebration. Take some of your favorite outdoor games, invite the friends, and have a cooler filled with icy drinks. On the grill, you can plan for things like corn on the cob that you have had to largely avoid while having your braces. It will make for a memorable afternoon!
- **Have a potluck dinner**. Have your friends each bring a dish people with braces have to take precaution with. This will give them the chance to learn a little more about what you went through, and it will be fun to see what options they come up with. Ask each of your guests to write down one comment about you with or without your braces. Your potluck will be filled with interesting dishes, laughs, and a good time!
- **Hit the spa**. What could be better then spending a couple of hours being pampered? Not much! Have a spa party for yourself, or invite a friend or two. Get a make-over, manicure, pedicure, massage, or whatever else you feel like

getting. Just pamper yourself for making it through your treatment. You will walk out feeling and looking great!

Doing some of the above things, such as chewing gum, may still not be good for your teeth or your body overall. But doing it on a special occasion, and not making a habit out of it, shouldn't do any harm.

Looking Ahead

Now that you have made it through wearing braces, you will find that you like to smile more, show off your beautiful teeth, and feel great! Having a celebration for getting your braces off is a great way to remember the day as something really special, include those you love, and start a new you!

There are many ways to celebrate. Think outside the box and determine what way will work best for you. Perhaps you want to have friends over, make it a family affair, or you just want to celebrate alone.

Whichever way you choose to do it, it will be a special day!

Epilogue:
You Had Questions, I Hope I've Provided the Answers

So, there you have it; two dozen of my patients' most popular questions. (For your convenience, I've included a handy FAQ directly after this Epilogue that summarizes most, if not all, of the questions we've just covered. Consider it a handy "Quick Reference" of sorts!)

The fact is, no book can ever answer EVERY question for every patient. Every case is unique, just as is every child's mouth. What I've tried to do is provide you with the basics and, hopefully, the confidence you'll need to ask further questions of your own orthodontist when and if they arise.

This is your child's mouth we're talking about here; never be afraid to open yours to make sure you're getting the answers you need! Now that you're armed with the answers to some of today's most frequently asked orthodontic questions, you can finally make the right decisions for your child's smile.

FAQs:

A Handy Resource Guide of Frequently Asked Questions and Orthodontic Terminology

What might happen if your child's mouth doesn't quite "fit"?
The fact is, the sooner you straighten your child's smile, the faster it will develop as it should; straight, clean and healthy!

Who are some famous faces who've worn braces?
Gwen Stefani. Prince Harry. Drew Barrymore. Tom Cruise. Dakota Fanning. Danny Glover.

Can I see what my child's straight teeth might look like first?
Yes! Digital pictures are often used to portray what the child's teeth might look like once the braces have been removed.

Will I be able to afford my child's braces?
Not only are most orthodontic procedures more affordable than ever, but insurance, payment plans and a variety of other financing options make this all but a moot point for most patients.

Will getting braces be painful for my child?
Not anymore; modern technology – and choosing the right orthodontist – can ensure that your child enjoys a pain-free orthodontic experience.

How much school will my child miss because of braces?
Not long, actually. After initial visits and barring the actual procedure itself, most visits and/or adjustments are routine and can take anywhere from 15 to 45 minutes.

Is it really such a big deal if my child has crooked teeth? Unfortunately, yes. Eroding, crooked or unaligned smiles can take time to happen, but the time to act is now. Orthodontic irregularities don't just heal on their own or "go away" if you ignore them.

What are some of the warning signs that my child might need to go to the orthodontist?
There are many, but here are a few of the most common: early or late loss of teeth, protruding teeth, grinding or clenching of teeth, speech difficulty, etc.

What kind of "side effects" can crooked teeth result in?
Some of the more frequent ones I see include headaches, toothaches, mouth breathing, chipped or worn down teeth, snoring and drooling.

What makes an orthodontist more qualified than a dentist? Orthodontists are dental specialists who have completed 2-3 years of additional education beyond dental school to learn the proper way to align teeth and jaws.

Why should I choose a specialist for my child's orthodontic care? Unique treatment requirements and otherwise difficult bite problems are common, everyday scenarios for your orthodontist. In the interest of receiving the most efficient and effective orthodontic treatment possible, choose an orthodontic specialist.

How do I know if my doctor is an orthodontist?
Only orthodontists can belong to the American Association of Orthodontists (AAO).

What is a treatment coordinator?
During your initial consultation(s), you will usually be assigned a patient contact person – we call this person a "treatment coordinator" in our office – with whom to schedule appointments, confer with

rescheduling and, of course, answer any and all questions you may have.

Why are follow-up visits important?
These are wonderful opportunities to either a.) ask questions you may have missed the first time or b.) get further details from your orthodontist him- or herself.

Why is early treatment so important?
Age seven is the earliest time your orthodontist can determine future jaw and tooth alignment. That's because, at the age of seven, your child's upper and lower permanent front teeth are developing. These teeth set the stage for future jaw position and serious problems can develop if they come into the wrong position.

Is there such a thing as a child being too old for braces? Actually, there is. Case in point: waiting to take your child to the orthodontist until they are 12 or 13 can be very risky.

What if I don't believe in early orthodontics?
Well, you're entitled to your opinion but, this is like saying you don't believe in the sun. You can hide from it, pretend it's not there or refuse to acknowledge it, but the simple fact remains. If you're not aware of the potential risks, you can get burnt.

Will my child actually need braces at seven?
Probably not. In the same breath I use to inform parents of the initial exam at age seven, I also mention that most children **will not need braces until 11-13 years of age**.

What is a crossbite?

When the upper and lower teeth grow at different rates, or times, or even when the lower jaw grows disproportionately with the upper jaw, something known as a "crossbite" can occur.

Where should I start to look for treatment if I'm concerned about my child's jaw development? If you suspect your child might have a crossbite, approach your family dentist about a recommendation to an orthodontist.

Why should I address a crossbite?
Crossbites can lead to pain, discomfort and lack of confidence as your child begins to feel insecure or even ostracized because of this very treatable, very normal series of jaw and teeth developments.

What is Invisalign?
The Invisalign system is the virtually invisible way to straighten your teeth and achieve the dazzling smile you've always dreamed of. Using advanced 3-D computer-imaging technology, Invisalign depicts your complete treatment plan, from the initial position of your teeth to the final desired position.

What are the primary benefits of Invisalign?
Like the word that inspired them, Invisalign aligners are practically clear; or as close to "invisible" as one can get. No one may even notice that you're wearing these virtually invisible "braces," making Invisalign a seamless fit with your lifestyle and day-to-day interactions with others.

How do I get started with Invisalign?
It's simple: just make an appointment with your local orthodontist for an initial consultation. Most doctors will offer a free initial consultation to see if you are a good candidate for Invisalign.

How will Invisalign effectively move my teeth?
Aligners are the foundation for, and work in concert with, the Invisalign system. Like brackets and arch wires are to braces, Invisalign aligners move teeth through the appropriate placement of controlled force on your child's teeth.

How many patients are being treated with Invisalign?
More than 1,000,000 patients worldwide have been treated with Invisalign. The number of Invisalign smiles grows daily.

Is Invisalign appropriate for my child?
Yes, because Invisalign now has a system designed specifically for teens!

How does Invisalign Teen work?
Aligners snap on your teeth easily. They are comfortable and practically invisible. Invisalign Teen allows for your growing permanent teeth and gently and continuously moves your teeth in small increments. Aligners are worn for about two weeks, then you swap them for a new pair.

Why are metal braces still so popular?
Well, for one thing, metal braces are very strong and can withstand most types of treatment. Today's metal braces are smaller, sleeker, and more polished than ever before.

Are so-called "clear braces" effective?

Ceramic braces are very strong and generally do not stain. Two popular brands are Clarity, made by 3M Unitek; and In-Ovation C, made by GAC. Adults like to choose ceramic because they "blend in" with the teeth and are less noticeable than metal. These are the type of braces actor Tom Cruise had.

Are clear braces appropriate for adults?

Absolutely! Adults of all ages can enjoy the same cosmetic and health benefits of properly aligned teeth with In-Ovation C system braces.

What are some of my payment options in addition to insurance?

One way many patients pay for their procedures is by utilizing the benefits of what is known as "Flex Spending," where their work matches their spending commitment.

What if my child has a "braces emergency" before or after office hours?

If you are experiencing an orthodontic emergency that can't wait for regular office hours, most orthodontic offices have a special number to call, either before, during or after business hours. If this information isn't given to you readily, check to see how your doctor's office handles emergencies.

Can a salt water rinse help?

Absolutely; warm saltwater rinses soothe the cheek lining, which can get aggravated by your child's braces.

How do I make a salt water rinse?

To make a salt water rinse, mix ½ teaspoon of table salt in one cup of warm water. Stir until the salt is completely dissolved. Gently swish about ¼ of the cup in your mouth for 30 seconds. Make sure you force the water over the areas that feel sore. Then spit the water into the sink. Repeat until the entire cup is gone.

What if my child plays sports and needs a mouth guard?

The best advice for patients or parents looking for a mouth guard can be obtained from your pediatrician, dentist, pediatric dentist, orthodontist or oral surgeon. All of these specialists are uniquely trained to offer customized advice in order to help you prevent a sports-related dental or facial injury.

What about brushing with braces?

Here are some simple tips you can share with your child for the best results when brushing with braces on:

- Brush your teeth with a medium nylon toothbrush after you eat and before bed.
- Brush, rinse, and look; if you find any areas that are not clean, brush them again.
- Brush your gums as you brush your teeth (massage and stimulate).
- If no toothpaste is available, brush without.
- If you are unable to brush, rinse your mouth vigorously with water.
- Replace your old toothbrush when it gets worn out.
- It is absolutely essential that you continue regular visits to your family dentist for checkups and cleanings throughout your orthodontic treatment!

What type of foods should my child avoid while wearing braces?

There are four main types of food your child should avoid while wearing braces: **hard foods** like ice, popcorn, peanut brittle, rock candy and corn on the cob; **sticky foods** like caramels, bubble gum, taffy and suckers; **chewy foods** like pizza crust, crusty breads, beef jerky and gummy bears; and **sugary foods and drinks**, like cake, ice cream, cookies, pie, candy and soda pop.

Why are retainers so important?
As we age, teeth naturally shift to the middle and crowd. Combined with late growth of the lower jaw, shifting of the teeth is expected following orthodontic treatment. Therefore, retainers are extremely important in the maintenance of your new smile following orthodontic treatment.

About the Author:
Dustin S. Burleson, DDS

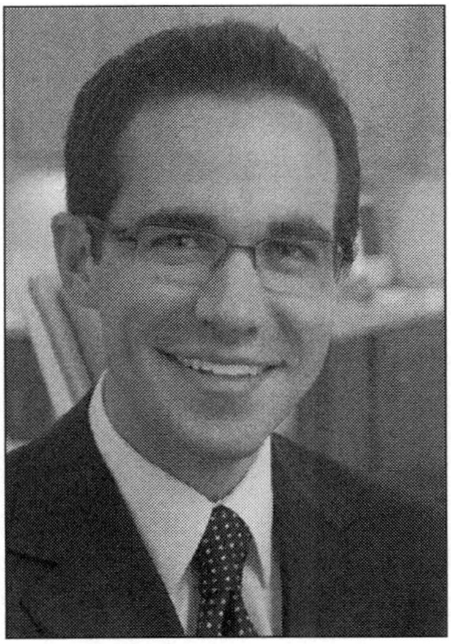

Doctor Burleson is an Assistant Clinical Professor in the Department of Orthodontics & Dentofacial Orthopedics at the University of Missouri - Kansas City School of Dentistry. He holds additional teaching affiliations with The Children's Mercy Hospital and Saint Luke's Hospital Cleft Palate and Craniofacial Teams. He maintains a private practice in Kansas City, Missouri, serves as the Director of The Leo H. Rheam Foundation for Cleft and Craniofacial Orthodontics, and is a ShareCare.com Expert in Dentistry and Orthodontics.

Dr. Burleson completed his undergraduate studies at the University of Missouri-Kansas City, where he earned a Bachelor of Arts in Biology, with distinction. He went on to receive his D.D.S. with distinction from the University of Missouri-Kansas City School of Dentistry, graduating with the highest academic standing in his class.

Dr. Burleson then completed his certificate of advanced graduate study in Orthodontics and Dentofacial Orthopedics at the UMKC School of Dentistry. Dr. Burleson continues to study the latest advances in his specialty through memberships in the following professional organizations:

American Board of Orthodontics
American Association of Orthodontists
American Cleft Palate-Craniofacial Association
American Dental Association
Missouri Dental Association
Greater Kansas City Dental Society
Charles H. Tweed International Foundation for Orthodontic Research

Dr. Burleson and his wife, Amy, reside in Kansas City, Missouri with their sons, Samuel, William and Benjamin.

Made in the USA
Monee, IL
05 November 2026

67380110R00065